Stage 3 Kidney Disease Diet Cookbook For Seniors

Cooking with Purpose: Flavorful Creations for Senior Kidney Diet Support

McDonnell B. Young

Table of Contents

Introduction

Last year, my grandfather, a spry and spirited 78-year-old, faced a daunting diagnosis: Stage 3 kidney disease. As a family, we were overwhelmed. The doctor explained the necessity of immediate dietary adjustments to manage his condition and slow its progression, but we were lost in a sea of vague guidelines and confusing advice—until we found the "Stage 3 Kidney Disease Diet Cookbook for Seniors."

When we first presented the cookbook to Grandpa Joe, his initial reaction was skepticism. He was set in his eating habits, and the idea of a diet overhaul was unappealing. But as he leafed through the book, something changed. The cookbook was not just a collection of recipes; it was a gateway to better health, specifically tailored for seniors like him.

The book was a treasure trove of easy-to-follow, kidney-friendly recipes crafted by dietitians specializing in renal health. Each recipe was designed to maintain the right balance of nutrients vital for kidney care, such as low sodium, controlled protein, and regulated potassium levels, all crucial for his stage of kidney disease.

What made this cookbook stand out was its understanding of its audience. It featured larger print, making it easy to read for aging eyes. The instructions were straightforward, considering the potential challenges seniors might face in the kitchen. It also included tips on meal planning and grocery shopping, which helped us as a family to support him effectively.

As weeks turned into months, Grandpa Joe found new favorites like the Apple and Cinnamon Porridge for breakfast and the Zesty Herb Chicken for dinner. He started looking forward to his meals instead of seeing them as a set of restrictions. The book didn't just prescribe; it inspired and educated. It included explanations about how each ingredient supports kidney health, which made him feel empowered and in control of his health.

Moreover, the cookbook came with guidance on modifying lifestyle habits that complement the dietary changes, providing a holistic approach to managing kidney disease. It encouraged gentle, senior-friendly exercises and offered advice on staying hydrated and managing other health conditions.

Seeing the transformation in my grandfather's health and spirits was profound. His energy levels improved, his lab results stabilized, and his doctor was impressed with the slowing progression of his kidney disease. This cookbook became our guide in a journey we initially thought we'd have to navigate in the dark.

I recommend the "Stage 3 Kidney Disease Diet Cookbook for Seniors" to anyone facing the challenges of kidney disease in their golden years. This guide is more than a cookbook—it's a companion that respects the unique needs of seniors, making a kidney-friendly diet achievable and enjoyable. It offers peace of mind, knowing you are doing everything possible to maintain your health and quality of life.

Every meal prepared from this cookbook is a testament to how proper nutrition can be both healing and delicious. It's an investment in health, a gesture of love, and a tool for empowerment. For families like mine, facing the uncertainty of kidney disease, this cookbook isn't just useful; it's essential.

Understanding Nutritional Needs and Restrictions

When dealing with Stage 3 kidney disease, managing dietary intake becomes crucial because the kidneys are less able to filter waste products and excess nutrients effectively. This cookbook specifically tailors its recipes to meet these needs by emphasizing low sodium, low potassium, and low phosphorus ingredients, which are essential to prevent further strain on the kidneys. By focusing on these dietary adjustments, the cookbook helps to stabilize kidney function and delay the progression of kidney disease, which is particularly important for seniors who are more susceptible to rapid declines in kidney health.

The recipes in the cookbook also consider protein intake, which is a critical aspect of a kidney-friendly diet. Excessive protein can cause a buildup of waste products in the blood, which can be harmful when your kidneys are compromised. However, it is also important not to consume too little protein, as it is vital for maintaining muscle mass, especially in the elderly. The cookbook strikes a balance by including moderate amounts of high-quality protein sources that are easier on the kidneys, ensuring that each meal delivers the right amount of protein.

Fluid intake is another important factor covered in the cookbook. While hydration is essential for good health, individuals with kidney disease often need to limit their fluid intake to prevent complications such as fluid overload, which can lead to swelling and high blood pressure. The cookbook offers creative ways to satisfy thirst and include moisture-rich foods that contribute to hydration without overloading the kidneys.

The selection of fruits and vegetables can be tricky for those with kidney disease due to the high potassium content in many common produce items. The cookbook provides lists of low-potassium fruits and vegetables and features them in its recipes. This allows for nutritional variety and the inclusion of essential vitamins and antioxidants in the diet, while still adhering to kidney-friendly guidelines.

Managing calcium and phosphorus intake is also vital, as kidney disease can affect the body's ability to regulate these minerals. This can lead to bone density issues and other metabolic complications. The cookbook includes recipes that are mindful of these minerals, using ingredients that help maintain a healthy balance. This is particularly important for seniors, who are already at risk for osteoporosis and other age-related conditions.

In addition to specific nutrient management, the cookbook addresses the overall caloric needs of seniors with kidney disease, which may differ from those of younger adults. Metabolic rates decrease with age, and the cookbook's recipes reflect appropriate portion sizes and calorie counts to maintain a healthy weight without burdening the kidneys.

Overall, the cookbook serves as an educational tool that guides seniors through the complexities of managing Stage 3 kidney disease through diet. It not only provides recipes but also helps seniors and their caregivers understand why each dietary adjustment is necessary, creating a sense of empowerment and control over their health. This comprehensive approach to dietary management can significantly improve the quality of life for seniors living with kidney disease, making each meal a calculated step towards better health.

Chapter 1: Breakfast – The Most Important Meal of the Day

Low Potassium Berry Smoothie

Ingredients:

- 1/2 cup of blueberries
- 1/2 cup of strawberries, sliced
- 1/4 cup of cranberries
- 1 cup of rice milk or almond milk (check labels to ensure they are low in potassium and phosphorus)
- 1 tablespoon of honey (optional, for sweetness)
- 1/2 cup of crushed ice or ice cubes

Instructions:

1. Combine blueberries, strawberries, cranberries, and milk in a blender.
2. Add honey if a sweeter taste is desired.
3. Blend on high until smooth.
4. Add ice and blend again until the smoothie reaches your preferred consistency.

Nutritional Information (per serving):

- Calories: 150
- Protein: 1 g
- Sodium: 50 mg
- Potassium: 200 mg
- Phosphorus: 60 mg

Serving Size: Makes 1 serving.

Cooking Time: 5 minutes.

Egg White Omelet with Mixed Veggies

Ingredients:

- 4 large egg whites
- 1/4 cup red bell pepper, diced
- 1/4 cup green bell pepper, diced
- 1/4 cup onion, finely chopped
- 1/4 cup mushrooms, sliced
- 1 tablespoon olive oil
- 1/4 teaspoon black pepper
- 1/4 teaspoon garlic powder
- Fresh parsley, chopped (optional, for garnish)

Instructions:

1. Heat the olive oil in a non-stick skillet over medium heat.
2. Add the onions, red bell pepper, green bell pepper, and mushrooms to the skillet. Sauté until the vegetables are tender, about 5-7 minutes.
3. In a bowl, whisk the egg whites with black pepper and garlic powder.
4. Pour the egg white mixture over the sautéed vegetables in the skillet.
5. Cook until the egg whites are set, about 3-4 minutes. Use a spatula to gently fold the omelet in half.
6. Cook for an additional 1-2 minutes to ensure the omelet is cooked through.

7. Slide the omelet onto a plate and garnish with fresh parsley if desired.

Nutritional Information:

- Calories: 110
- Protein: 12g
- Carbohydrates: 4g
- Fat: 5g
- Sodium: 140mg
- Potassium: 220mg
- Phosphorus: 30mg

Serving Size:

- 1 omelet (serves 1)

Cooking Time:

- Total: 15 minutes

Apple and Cinnamon Oatmeal

Ingredient:

- 1/2 cup rolled oats
- 1 cup water
- 1/2 cup unsweetened almond milk
- 1 small apple, peeled, cored, and diced
- 1/2 teaspoon ground cinnamon
- 1 teaspoon honey (optional)
- A pinch of salt

Instructions:

1. In a medium saucepan, bring the water to a boil.
2. Add the rolled oats and reduce the heat to a simmer.
3. Stir in the diced apple and ground cinnamon.
4. Cook for about 5-7 minutes, stirring occasionally, until the oats are tender and the mixture thickens.
5. Add the unsweetened almond milk and cook for another 2-3 minutes.
6. Remove from heat and let it sit for a minute before serving.
7. Drizzle with honey if desired.

Nutritional Information:

- Calories: 220
- Protein: 5g
- Carbohydrates: 40g

- Fiber: 6g
- Sugars: 12g
- Sodium: 60mg
- Potassium: 200mg
- Phosphorus: 100mg

Serving Size:

- Serves 1

Cooking Time:

- 15 minutes

Buckwheat Pancakes with Blueberries

Ingredient:

- 1 cup buckwheat flour
- 1 tablespoon sugar
- 1 teaspoon baking powder
- 1/2 teaspoon baking soda
- 1/4 teaspoon salt
- 1 cup buttermilk (or a kidney-friendly alternative)
- 1 large egg
- 2 tablespoons unsalted butter, melted
- 1/2 cup fresh or frozen blueberries

Instructions:

1. In a large bowl, whisk together the buckwheat flour, sugar, baking powder, baking soda, and salt.
2. In a separate bowl, whisk the buttermilk and egg until well combined.
3. Pour the wet ingredients into the dry ingredients and mix until just combined. Do not overmix.
4. Gently fold in the melted butter and blueberries.
5. Heat a non-stick skillet or griddle over medium heat. Lightly grease with a small amount of unsalted butter or oil.
6. Pour 1/4 cup of batter onto the skillet for each pancake. Cook until bubbles form on the surface and the edges look set, about 2-3 minutes.

7. Flip the pancakes and cook for an additional 2-3 minutes until golden brown and cooked through.

8. Serve warm, optionally with a small drizzle of pure maple syrup or a sprinkle of powdered sugar.

Nutritional Information:

- Calories: 180 per serving
- Protein: 5g
- Carbohydrates: 28g
- Dietary Fiber: 4g
- Sugars: 6g
- Fat: 6g
- Saturated Fat: 3g
- Sodium: 150mg
- Potassium: 150mg
- Phosphorus: 80mg

Serving Size:

- Makes 4 servings (2 pancakes per serving)

Cooking Time:

- Preparation: 10 minutes
- Cooking: 15 minutes
- Total: 25 minutes

Almond Milk Rice Pudding

Ingredients:

- 1 cup cooked white rice
- 1 cup unsweetened almond milk
- 2 tablespoons sugar or sugar substitute
- 1 teaspoon vanilla extract
- 1/4 teaspoon ground cinnamon
- 1/4 cup raisins (optional)

Instructions:

1. In a medium saucepan, combine the cooked white rice and almond milk.
2. Cook over medium heat, stirring frequently, until the mixture begins to thicken, about 10-15 minutes.
3. Add the sugar, vanilla extract, and ground cinnamon, stirring well to combine.
4. If using raisins, stir them in and continue to cook for an additional 5 minutes, or until the pudding reaches your desired consistency.
5. Remove from heat and let it cool slightly before serving. The pudding will thicken further as it cools.

Nutritional Information:

- Calories: 150
- Protein: 3 grams

- Carbohydrates: 30 grams
- Dietary Fiber: 1 gram
- Sugar: 12 grams
- Fat: 2 grams
- Sodium: 45 milligrams
- Potassium: 50 milligrams
- Phosphorus: 40 milligrams

Serving Size: 1/2 cup

Cooking Time: 20 minutes

Toasted Whole Grain Bread with Avocado Spread

Ingredients:

- 2 slices of whole grain bread
- 1 ripe avocado
- 1 tablespoon lemon juice
- 1/4 teaspoon garlic powder
- 1/4 teaspoon salt (optional)
- A pinch of black pepper
- Fresh cilantro or parsley for garnish (optional)

Instructions:

1. Toast the slices of whole grain bread to your desired level of crispiness.
2. While the bread is toasting, cut the avocado in half, remove the pit, and scoop the flesh into a small bowl.
3. Add the lemon juice, garlic powder, salt (if using), and black pepper to the avocado. Mash together with a fork until smooth and well-mixed.
4. Once the bread is toasted, spread the avocado mixture evenly over each slice.
5. Garnish with fresh cilantro or parsley if desired.
6. Serve immediately.

Nutritional Information (per serving):

- Calories: 220
- Protein: 4 grams
- Carbohydrates: 25 grams
- Fiber: 10 grams
- Fat: 12 grams
- Sodium: 150 mg (without added salt)

Serving Size:

- 1 serving (2 slices of toast)

Cooking Time:

- Preparation: 10 minutes
- Cooking: 5 minutes
- Total: 15 minutes

Low Sodium Cottage Cheese with Pineapple

Ingredients:

- 1 cup low sodium cottage cheese
- 1/2 cup fresh pineapple chunks
- 1 teaspoon honey (optional)
- A sprinkle of cinnamon (optional)

Instructions:

1. Place the cottage cheese in a bowl.
2. Add the pineapple chunks on top of the cottage cheese.
3. Drizzle with honey if desired.
4. Sprinkle with cinnamon if desired.
5. Mix gently and serve immediately.

Nutritional Information:

- Calories: 150
- Protein: 14g
- Carbohydrates: 16g
- Fat: 2g
- Sodium: 90mg
- Potassium: 180mg
- Phosphorus: 120mg

Serving Size:

- Serves 1

Cooking Time:

- Preparation time: 5 minutes

Cream of Wheat with a Hint of Honey

Ingredients:

- 1/4 cup Cream of Wheat
- 1 cup water
- 1 teaspoon honey
- 1/4 teaspoon vanilla extract
- Dash of cinnamon (optional)
- A pinch of salt (optional)

Instructions:

1. In a small saucepan, bring the water to a boil.
2. Gradually stir in the Cream of Wheat, reducing the heat to low.
3. Cook, stirring constantly, for about 2-3 minutes or until the mixture thickens.
4. Remove from heat and stir in the honey and vanilla extract.
5. Add a dash of cinnamon for extra flavor if desired.
6. Serve warm.

Nutritional Information:

- Calories: 80
- Protein: 3g
- Carbohydrates: 18g
- Dietary Fiber: 1g
- Sugars: 4g
- Fat: 0.5g

- Sodium: 5mg
- Potassium: 35mg
- Phosphorus: 25mg

Serving Size: 1 serving

Cooking Time: 5 minutes

Greek Yogurt Parfait with Raspberries

Ingredient:

- 1 cup plain Greek yogurt (low-fat or non-fat)

- 1/2 cup fresh raspberries

- 1 tablespoon honey

- 1/4 cup low-sugar granola

- 1 teaspoon chia seeds

Instructions:

1. Spoon the Greek yogurt into a bowl or parfait glass.

2. Layer the fresh raspberries on top of the yogurt.

3. Drizzle the honey over the raspberries.

4. Sprinkle the low-sugar granola over the honey.

5. Top with chia seeds for added texture and nutrition.

Nutritional Information:

- Calories: 200

- Protein: 12g

- Carbohydrates: 28g

- Sugars: 18g

- Fat: 4g

- Sodium: 50mg

- Potassium: 150mg

- Phosphorus: 130mg

Serving Size:

- 1 serving

Cooking Time:

- 5 minutes

Homemade Muesli with No Added Sugar

Ingredient:

- 1 cup rolled oats
- 1/4 cup unsweetened dried cranberries
- 1/4 cup unsweetened coconut flakes
- 1/4 cup raw pumpkin seeds
- 1/4 cup chopped almonds
- 1/4 teaspoon ground cinnamon
- 1 cup unsweetened almond milk (or other kidney-friendly milk substitute)

Instructions:

1. In a large bowl, combine rolled oats, dried cranberries, coconut flakes, pumpkin seeds, chopped almonds, and ground cinnamon. Mix well.
2. Store the muesli mixture in an airtight container.
3. When ready to serve, scoop 1/2 cup of the muesli mixture into a bowl.
4. Pour 1/2 cup of unsweetened almond milk over the muesli and stir to combine.
5. Let it sit for a few minutes to allow the oats to soften.
6. Serve immediately or refrigerate overnight for a softer texture.

Nutritional Information (per serving):

- Calories: 220
- Protein: 6g
- Carbohydrates: 35g
- Fiber: 6g
- Sugars: 6g (natural sugars from cranberries)
- Fat: 8g
- Sodium: 10mg
- Potassium: 220mg
- Phosphorus: 90mg

Serving Size:

- 1/2 cup muesli mixture with 1/2 cup almond milk

Cooking Time:

- Preparation: 10 minutes
- Resting (optional): Overnight (for softer texture)

Chapter 2: Lunch – Fueling the Day

Grilled Chicken Salad with Olive Oil Dressing

Ingredients:

- 1 boneless, skinless chicken breast (about 4 ounces)
- 1 tablespoon olive oil
- 1 teaspoon dried oregano
- 1 cup mixed salad greens (such as romaine, arugula, and spinach)
- 1/2 cup cherry tomatoes, halved
- 1/4 cup cucumber, sliced
- 1/4 red bell pepper, thinly sliced
- 1 tablespoon unsalted sunflower seeds
- Juice of 1/2 lemon
- 1 tablespoon balsamic vinegar
- 1 garlic clove, minced
- Freshly ground black pepper to taste

Instructions:

1. Preheat the grill to medium-high heat. Season the chicken breast with oregano and a pinch of black pepper.
2. Brush the grill with olive oil to prevent sticking. Grill the chicken for about 5-6 minutes per side, or until fully cooked and the internal temperature reaches 165°F.
3. Remove the chicken from the grill and let it rest for a few minutes before slicing it into thin strips.
4. In a large bowl, combine the salad greens, cherry tomatoes, cucumber, and red bell pepper.
5. In a small bowl, whisk together the lemon juice, balsamic vinegar, minced garlic, and remaining olive oil to make the dressing.
6. Toss the salad with the dressing, ensuring all ingredients are evenly coated.
7. Top the salad with the grilled chicken slices and sprinkle with unsalted sunflower seeds.
8. Serve immediately.

Nutritional Information:

- Calories: 280
- Protein: 25g
- Carbohydrates: 8g
- Dietary Fiber: 2g
- Sugars: 4g
- Fat: 16g
- Saturated Fat: 2g

- Sodium: 75mg
- Potassium: 420mg
- Phosphorus: 210mg

Serving Size:

1 serving (entire recipe)

Cooking Time:

20 minutes

Roasted Turkey and Quinoa Wrap

Ingredient:

- 1/2 cup cooked quinoa (cooled)
- 1/4 cup finely chopped cucumber
- 1/4 cup finely chopped red bell pepper
- 1/4 cup finely chopped fresh parsley
- 1 tablespoon olive oil
- 1 tablespoon lemon juice
- 1/4 teaspoon ground black pepper
- 4 ounces thinly sliced roasted turkey breast (low sodium)
- 2 large whole wheat tortillas
- 1/2 cup mixed salad greens

Instructions:

1. In a medium bowl, combine the cooked quinoa, cucumber, red bell pepper, and parsley.

2. In a small bowl, whisk together the olive oil, lemon juice, and ground black pepper. Pour this dressing over the quinoa mixture and toss to coat.

3. Lay out the whole wheat tortillas on a clean surface. Place 2 ounces of roasted turkey breast on each tortilla.

4. Evenly distribute the quinoa mixture over the turkey slices.

5. Top with mixed salad greens.

6. Roll up each tortilla tightly and slice in half if desired.

7. Serve immediately or wrap in foil for a portable lunch option.

Nutritional Information:

- Calories: 320 per wrap
- Protein: 22 grams
- Carbohydrates: 35 grams
- Fiber: 6 grams
- Fat: 10 grams
- Sodium: 320 milligrams
- Potassium: 450 milligrams
- Phosphorus: 220 milligrams

Serving Size:

- 1 wrap (half of the recipe)

Cooking Time:

- Preparation: 20 minutes
- No additional cooking time required

Vegetable Soup with No-Salt Added Broth

Ingredient:

- 1 tablespoon olive oil
- 1 small onion, diced
- 2 cloves garlic, minced
- 2 medium carrots, diced
- 2 celery stalks, diced
- 1 zucchini, diced
- 1 cup green beans, cut into 1-inch pieces
- 1 cup cabbage, shredded
- 4 cups no-salt-added vegetable broth
- 1 teaspoon dried thyme
- 1 teaspoon dried basil
- 1/2 teaspoon black pepper
- 1 cup diced tomatoes (no salt added)
- 1/2 cup frozen peas
- Fresh parsley for garnish (optional)

Instructions:

1. Heat the olive oil in a large pot over medium heat. Add the onion and garlic, sautéing until they are soft and fragrant, about 5 minutes.

2. Add the carrots, celery, zucchini, green beans, and cabbage to the pot. Cook for another 5-7 minutes, stirring occasionally.

3. Pour in the no-salt-added vegetable broth and add the dried thyme, dried basil, and black pepper. Bring the soup to a boil, then reduce the heat to a simmer.

4. Add the diced tomatoes and let the soup simmer for about 20 minutes, or until the vegetables are tender.

5. Stir in the frozen peas and cook for an additional 5 minutes.

6. Serve hot, garnished with fresh parsley if desired.

Nutritional Information (per serving):

- Calories: 110
- Protein: 3g
- Carbohydrates: 18g
- Dietary Fiber: 5g
- Sugars: 7g
- Fat: 4g
- Saturated Fat: 0.5g
- Sodium: 35mg
- Potassium: 420mg
- Phosphorus: 55mg

Serving Size:

- Serves 4

Cooking Time:

- Total: 45 minutes

Tuna Salad with Low Sodium Mayo

Ingredients:

- 1 can (5 oz) low sodium tuna, drained
- 2 tablespoons low sodium mayonnaise
- 1 tablespoon plain Greek yogurt
- 1 celery stalk, finely chopped
- 1/4 cup red bell pepper, finely chopped
- 1 tablespoon fresh lemon juice
- 1 teaspoon Dijon mustard
- 1/4 teaspoon ground black pepper
- 1 tablespoon fresh parsley, chopped

Instructions:

1. In a medium bowl, combine the low sodium mayonnaise, Greek yogurt, lemon juice, Dijon mustard, and ground black pepper. Mix until smooth.
2. Add the drained tuna, chopped celery, red bell pepper, and fresh parsley to the bowl. Mix until all ingredients are well incorporated.
3. Taste and adjust seasoning if necessary, keeping in mind the low sodium requirement.
4. Serve the tuna salad on a bed of lettuce, with whole-grain crackers, or in a low sodium whole wheat pita.

Nutritional Information:

- Calories: 150 per serving
- Protein: 20g
- Carbohydrates: 3g
- Fat: 5g
- Sodium: 120mg
- Potassium: 200mg
- Phosphorus: 150mg

Serving Size:

- Makes 2 servings

Cooking Time:

- Preparation time: 15 minutes
- Cooking time: None

Baked Salmon with Herb Dressing

Ingredients:

- 4 oz salmon fillet
- 1 tbsp olive oil
- 1 tbsp fresh lemon juice
- 1 tbsp fresh parsley, chopped
- 1 clove garlic, minced
- 1 tsp dried oregano
- 1/4 tsp ground black pepper
- 1/2 cup green beans, steamed
- 1/2 cup carrot slices, steamed

Instructions:

1. Preheat the oven to 375°F (190°C).
2. Place the salmon fillet on a baking sheet lined with parchment paper.
3. In a small bowl, mix olive oil, lemon juice, parsley, garlic, oregano, and black pepper.
4. Brush the herb mixture evenly over the salmon fillet.
5. Bake the salmon in the preheated oven for 15-20 minutes, or until the fish flakes easily with a fork.
6. While the salmon is baking, steam the green beans and carrot slices until tender.
7. Serve the baked salmon with the steamed vegetables on the side.

Nutritional Information:

- Calories: 250
- Protein: 23g
- Carbohydrates: 10g
- Fat: 12g
- Sodium: 90mg
- Potassium: 450mg
- Phosphorus: 200mg

Serving Size: 1 salmon fillet with 1 cup of vegetables

Cooking Time: 30 minutes

Stir-Fried Tofu with Veggies in Olive Oil

Ingredient:

- 1 block of firm tofu, drained and cubed
- 2 tablespoons olive oil
- 1 cup broccoli florets
- 1 red bell pepper, sliced
- 1 small zucchini, sliced
- 1/2 cup snap peas
- 2 cloves garlic, minced
- 1 tablespoon low-sodium soy sauce
- 1 tablespoon rice vinegar
- 1/2 teaspoon ground ginger
- Fresh parsley for garnish (optional)

Instructions:

1. Heat 1 tablespoon of olive oil in a large skillet over medium heat.
2. Add the cubed tofu and cook until golden brown on all sides, about 5-7 minutes. Remove from the skillet and set aside.
3. In the same skillet, add the remaining tablespoon of olive oil.
4. Add the minced garlic and cook until fragrant, about 1 minute.
5. Add the broccoli, red bell pepper, zucchini, and snap peas to the skillet. Stir-fry for 5-7 minutes until the vegetables are tender-crisp.

6. Return the tofu to the skillet and stir to combine.

7. In a small bowl, mix the low-sodium soy sauce, rice vinegar, and ground ginger. Pour the mixture over the tofu and vegetables.

8. Stir well to coat everything evenly. Cook for another 2-3 minutes to heat through.

9. Remove from heat and garnish with fresh parsley if desired.

10. Serve immediately.

Nutritional Information:

- Calories: 250
- Protein: 15g
- Carbohydrates: 20g
- Dietary Fiber: 5g
- Total Fat: 12g
- Saturated Fat: 2g
- Sodium: 150mg
- Potassium: 400mg
- Phosphorus: 150mg

Serving Size: 1 cup

Cooking Time: 20 minutes

Beef Stew with Potatoes and Carrots

Ingredients:

- 1 pound lean beef stew meat, cut into 1-inch cubes
- 2 medium potatoes, peeled and cubed
- 3 large carrots, peeled and sliced
- 1 large onion, chopped
- 2 cloves garlic, minced
- 4 cups low-sodium beef broth
- 1 tablespoon olive oil
- 1 teaspoon dried thyme
- 1 teaspoon dried rosemary
- 1 bay leaf
- 1/4 teaspoon black pepper

Instructions:

1. In a large pot, heat the olive oil over medium heat. Add the beef and cook until browned on all sides, about 5-7 minutes.
2. Remove the beef from the pot and set it aside. Add the onion and garlic to the pot and sauté until the onion is translucent, about 3-4 minutes.
3. Return the beef to the pot and add the low-sodium beef broth, dried thyme, dried rosemary, bay leaf, and black pepper. Stir to combine.
4. Bring the mixture to a boil, then reduce the heat to low. Cover and simmer for 1 hour, stirring occasionally.

5. Add the potatoes and carrots to the pot. Cover and continue to simmer for an additional 30 minutes, or until the vegetables are tender.

6. Remove the bay leaf before serving.

Nutritional Information:

- Calories: 250 per serving
- Protein: 18g
- Carbohydrates: 25g
- Dietary Fiber: 4g
- Sugars: 5g
- Fat: 8g
- Saturated Fat: 2.5g
- Sodium: 150mg
- Potassium: 600mg
- Phosphorus: 200mg

Serving Size:

4 servings

Cooking Time:

1 hour and 45 minutes

Pasta Salad with Cherry Tomatoes and Basil

Ingredient:

- 2 cups of cooked pasta (preferably whole wheat or low-protein pasta)
- 1 cup of cherry tomatoes, halved
- 1/4 cup of fresh basil leaves, chopped
- 2 tablespoons of extra virgin olive oil
- 1 tablespoon of red wine vinegar
- 1 teaspoon of minced garlic
- Salt-free seasoning blend to taste
- Freshly ground black pepper to taste

Instructions:

1. Cook the pasta according to the package instructions. Drain and rinse under cold water to cool.
2. In a large mixing bowl, combine the cooked pasta, cherry tomatoes, and chopped basil.
3. In a small bowl, whisk together the olive oil, red wine vinegar, and minced garlic.
4. Pour the dressing over the pasta mixture and toss to coat evenly.
5. Season with a salt-free seasoning blend and freshly ground black pepper to taste.
6. Chill in the refrigerator for at least 30 minutes before serving to allow the flavors to meld.

Nutritional Information:

- Calories: 220 per serving
- Protein: 5g
- Carbohydrates: 30g
- Fat: 10g
- Sodium: 15mg
- Potassium: 200mg
- Phosphorus: 70mg

Serving Size:

- 1 cup

Cooking Time:

- 20 minutes (plus 30 minutes chilling time)

Egg Salad on Whole Wheat Bread

Ingredient:

- 2 large eggs
- 2 tablespoons mayonnaise (low-sodium)
- 1 teaspoon Dijon mustard
- 1 tablespoon chopped fresh parsley
- 1 tablespoon chopped celery
- 1 tablespoon chopped onion
- 1/8 teaspoon black pepper
- 2 slices whole wheat bread (low-sodium)
- Lettuce leaves (optional)

Instructions:

1. Place the eggs in a saucepan and cover with cold water. Bring to a boil over medium-high heat.
2. Once boiling, reduce heat to low and simmer for 10-12 minutes.
3. Remove the eggs from heat, drain, and place in cold water to cool.
4. Peel the eggs and chop them into small pieces.
5. In a medium bowl, combine chopped eggs, mayonnaise, Dijon mustard, parsley, celery, onion, and black pepper. Mix well.
6. Spread the egg salad evenly over one slice of whole wheat bread.
7. Top with lettuce leaves if desired, then place the second slice of bread on top.

8. Cut the sandwich in half and serve immediately.

Nutritional Information (per serving):

- Calories: 250
- Protein: 12g
- Carbohydrates: 24g
- Total Fat: 12g
- Saturated Fat: 2g
- Cholesterol: 210mg
- Sodium: 320mg
- Potassium: 150mg
- Phosphorus: 160mg

Serving Size:

- 1 sandwich (serves 1)

Cooking Time:

- 20 minutes

Vegetable and Bean Chili

Ingredients:

- 1 tablespoon olive oil
- 1 medium onion, chopped
- 2 cloves garlic, minced
- 1 red bell pepper, chopped
- 1 yellow bell pepper, chopped
- 2 carrots, peeled and diced
- 1 zucchini, diced
- 1 can (15 ounces) low-sodium kidney beans, drained and rinsed
- 1 can (15 ounces) low-sodium black beans, drained and rinsed
- 1 can (15 ounces) no-salt-added diced tomatoes
- 2 cups low-sodium vegetable broth
- 1 tablespoon chili powder
- 1 teaspoon ground cumin
- 1/2 teaspoon dried oregano
- 1/4 teaspoon black pepper
- 1/4 teaspoon paprika
- Fresh cilantro for garnish (optional)

Instructions:

1. Heat olive oil in a large pot over medium heat.
2. Add chopped onion and garlic; sauté until fragrant and translucent, about 5 minutes.

3. Add bell peppers, carrots, and zucchini; cook until vegetables are tender, about 8 minutes.

4. Stir in the kidney beans, black beans, diced tomatoes, and vegetable broth.

5. Add chili powder, cumin, oregano, black pepper, and paprika.

6. Bring to a boil, then reduce heat and simmer for 30 minutes, stirring occasionally.

7. Adjust seasoning if necessary, and garnish with fresh cilantro if desired.

Nutritional Information:

- Calories: 210 per serving
- Protein: 8 grams
- Carbohydrates: 37 grams
- Dietary Fiber: 10 grams
- Sugars: 9 grams
- Fat: 3.5 grams
- Sodium: 150 milligrams
- Potassium: 580 milligrams
- Phosphorus: 120 milligrams

Serving Size: 1 cup

Cooking Time: 45 minutes

Chapter 3: Dinner – Ending the Day Right

Grilled Pork Tenderloin with a Spice Rub

Ingredients:

- 1 pound pork tenderloin
- 1 tablespoon olive oil
- 1 teaspoon garlic powder
- 1 teaspoon onion powder
- 1 teaspoon smoked paprika
- 1/2 teaspoon dried thyme
- 1/2 teaspoon dried oregano
- 1/2 teaspoon ground black pepper
- 1/4 teaspoon salt (optional or adjusted to taste)

Instructions:

1. Preheat the grill to medium-high heat.
2. In a small bowl, mix together the garlic powder, onion powder, smoked paprika, thyme, oregano, black pepper, and salt (if using).
3. Rub the pork tenderloin with olive oil to coat it evenly.
4. Apply the spice mixture all over the pork tenderloin, ensuring it is well-coated.

5. Place the pork tenderloin on the preheated grill.

6. Grill the pork for about 15-20 minutes, turning occasionally, until the internal temperature reaches 145°F (63°C) for medium-rare, or cook longer if desired.

7. Remove the pork from the grill and let it rest for 5 minutes before slicing.

Nutritional Information (per serving):

- Calories: 200
- Protein: 26 grams
- Carbohydrates: 2 grams
- Dietary Fiber: 1 gram
- Total Fat: 10 grams
- Saturated Fat: 2 grams
- Sodium: 150 milligrams
- Potassium: 400 milligrams
- Phosphorus: 210 milligrams

Serving Size:

- Serves 4

Cooking Time:

- Preparation: 10 minutes
- Cooking: 20 minutes

Lemon Baked Cod with Green Beans

Ingredients

- 4 (4-ounce) cod fillets
- 1 tablespoon olive oil
- 1 lemon, thinly sliced
- 1 teaspoon dried thyme
- 1 teaspoon dried oregano
- 2 garlic cloves, minced
- 1 pound fresh green beans, trimmed
- 1/4 teaspoon salt
- 1/4 teaspoon black pepper

Instructions

1. Preheat your oven to 400°F (200°C).
2. Place the cod fillets in a baking dish and drizzle with olive oil.
3. Arrange lemon slices over the cod fillets.
4. Sprinkle thyme, oregano, and minced garlic evenly over the fish.
5. Place the green beans around the fish in the baking dish.
6. Season the entire dish with salt and pepper.
7. Cover the baking dish with aluminum foil and bake for 20-25 minutes, or until the fish flakes easily with a fork and the green beans are tender.
8. Remove the foil for the last 5 minutes of baking to allow the fish to lightly brown.

Nutritional Information

- Calories: 200 per serving
- Protein: 24 grams
- Carbohydrates: 8 grams
- Dietary Fiber: 4 grams
- Total Fat: 7 grams
- Sodium: 150 milligrams
- Potassium: 400 milligrams
- Phosphorus: 200 milligrams

Serving Size

- 1 fillet with 1/4 of the green beans

Cooking Time

- Total: 30 minutes

Stir-Fried Shrimp and Broccoli

Ingredient:

- 1 lb large shrimp, peeled and deveined
- 2 cups broccoli florets
- 1 tablespoon olive oil
- 2 cloves garlic, minced
- 1 tablespoon low-sodium soy sauce
- 1 teaspoon grated fresh ginger
- 1/2 cup low-sodium chicken broth
- 1 teaspoon cornstarch mixed with 2 tablespoons water
- 1 teaspoon sesame oil
- 1/4 teaspoon black pepper

Instructions:

1. Heat the olive oil in a large skillet or wok over medium-high heat.
2. Add the garlic and ginger, stirring constantly for about 30 seconds until fragrant.
3. Add the shrimp and cook for 2-3 minutes, turning until they turn pink and are cooked through. Remove the shrimp from the skillet and set aside.
4. In the same skillet, add the broccoli florets and cook for 3-4 minutes until they are tender-crisp.
5. Return the shrimp to the skillet with the broccoli.

6. Add the low-sodium soy sauce and low-sodium chicken broth, stirring to combine.

7. Stir in the cornstarch mixture and cook for another 1-2 minutes until the sauce has thickened.

8. Drizzle with sesame oil and sprinkle with black pepper before serving.

Nutritional Information:

- Calories: 220 per serving
- Protein: 28g
- Carbohydrates: 8g
- Fat: 8g
- Sodium: 200mg
- Potassium: 400mg
- Phosphorus: 250mg

Serving Size:

- Serves 4

Cooking Time:

- Total time: 20 minutes

Vegetable Lasagna with Ricotta Cheese

Ingredient:

- 1 package (9 ounces) no-boil lasagna noodles
- 2 cups low-sodium marinara sauce
- 1 medium zucchini, thinly sliced
- 1 medium yellow squash, thinly sliced
- 1 cup baby spinach, chopped
- 1 cup ricotta cheese (low-fat)
- 1 cup shredded mozzarella cheese (low-sodium)
- 1/2 cup grated Parmesan cheese (optional)
- 2 tablespoons olive oil
- 1 teaspoon dried basil
- 1 teaspoon dried oregano
- 1/2 teaspoon garlic powder
- 1/2 teaspoon onion powder

Instructions:

1. Preheat the oven to 375°F (190°C).
2. In a large skillet, heat olive oil over medium heat. Add zucchini and yellow squash, cooking until slightly tender, about 5 minutes.
3. In a medium bowl, combine ricotta cheese, dried basil, dried oregano, garlic powder, and onion powder.
4. Spread a thin layer of marinara sauce on the bottom of a 9x13 inch baking dish.
5. Place a layer of lasagna noodles over the sauce.

6. Spread half of the ricotta mixture over the noodles, then layer with half of the cooked zucchini and squash, and a handful of chopped spinach.

7. Add another layer of marinara sauce, then repeat the layers with noodles, ricotta mixture, vegetables, and sauce.

8. Finish with a final layer of lasagna noodles and marinara sauce. Sprinkle mozzarella cheese on top.

9. Cover with aluminum foil and bake for 30 minutes.

10. Remove the foil and bake an additional 15 minutes, or until the cheese is bubbly and slightly browned.

11. Let the lasagna cool for 10 minutes before serving.

Nutritional Information:

- Calories: 280 per serving
- Protein: 15g
- Carbohydrates: 35g
- Dietary Fiber: 4g
- Sugars: 8g
- Total Fat: 10g
- Saturated Fat: 4g
- Sodium: 200mg
- Potassium: 350mg
- Phosphorus: 180mg

Serving Size:

- 1 piece (approximately 1/9 of the lasagna)

Cooking Time:

- Total: 55 minutes (40 minutes baking, 15 minutes cooling)

Chicken Stir Fry with Bell Peppers

Ingredients:

- 1 lb skinless, boneless chicken breast, sliced into thin strips
- 1 red bell pepper, sliced
- 1 yellow bell pepper, sliced
- 1 green bell pepper, sliced
- 1 small onion, sliced
- 2 cloves garlic, minced
- 1 tablespoon olive oil
- 2 tablespoons low-sodium soy sauce
- 1 tablespoon rice vinegar
- 1 teaspoon ground ginger
- 1/4 teaspoon black pepper
- 1/2 cup low-sodium chicken broth
- 2 cups cooked white rice (optional)

Instructions:

1. Heat olive oil in a large skillet or wok over medium-high heat.
2. Add the sliced chicken breast and cook until browned and cooked through, about 5-7 minutes. Remove chicken from the skillet and set aside.
3. In the same skillet, add the minced garlic and sliced onion. Cook until the onion becomes translucent, about 3 minutes.
4. Add the sliced bell peppers to the skillet and stir-fry for another 5 minutes until they are tender but still crisp.

5. Return the chicken to the skillet. Add the low-sodium soy sauce, rice vinegar, ground ginger, black pepper, and low-sodium chicken broth. Stir well to combine.

6. Cook for an additional 2-3 minutes, allowing the flavors to meld together and the sauce to thicken slightly.

7. Serve the stir fry over cooked white rice if desired, ensuring portion control to maintain appropriate protein intake.

Nutritional Information (per serving, without rice):

- Calories: 220
- Protein: 28g
- Carbohydrates: 9g
- Dietary Fiber: 2g
- Sugars: 4g
- Fat: 8g
- Saturated Fat: 1.5g
- Sodium: 210mg
- Potassium: 450mg
- Phosphorus: 230mg

Serving Size:

- Serves 4

Cooking Time:

- 25 minutes

Baked Trout with Lemon and Herbs

Ingredients:

- 4 trout fillets (about 4-6 ounces each)
- 2 tablespoons olive oil
- 1 lemon, thinly sliced
- 2 tablespoons fresh parsley, chopped
- 1 tablespoon fresh dill, chopped
- 2 cloves garlic, minced
- Salt substitute (optional)
- Freshly ground black pepper to taste

Instructions:

1. Preheat the oven to 375°F (190°C).
2. Rinse the trout fillets under cold water and pat dry with paper towels.
3. Place the fillets in a baking dish, skin side down.
4. Drizzle olive oil evenly over the fillets.
5. Arrange the lemon slices on top of the fillets.
6. Sprinkle parsley, dill, and minced garlic over the fillets.
7. Add salt substitute and freshly ground black pepper to taste.
8. Cover the baking dish with aluminum foil.
9. Bake in the preheated oven for 20-25 minutes, or until the fish flakes easily with a fork.
10. Remove from the oven and let it rest for a few minutes before serving.

Nutritional Information:

- Calories: 220 per serving
- Protein: 28g
- Carbohydrates: 2g
- Total Fat: 11g
- Saturated Fat: 2g
- Cholesterol: 70mg
- Sodium: 60mg
- Potassium: 490mg
- Phosphorus: 210mg

Serving Size: 1 fillet (4-6 ounces)

Cooking Time: 30 minutes (including preparation)

Roast Beef with Mashed Cauliflower

Ingredients:

- 1 pound lean beef roast
- 1 head of cauliflower, chopped
- 2 tablespoons olive oil
- 1 teaspoon garlic powder
- 1 teaspoon dried thyme
- 1/2 teaspoon black pepper
- 1/4 teaspoon salt
- 1/4 cup low-sodium beef broth
- 1 tablespoon unsalted butter
- 2 tablespoons fresh parsley, chopped

Instructions:

1. Preheat the oven to 375°F.

2. Rub the beef roast with olive oil, garlic powder, dried thyme, black pepper, and salt.

3. Place the roast in a baking dish and pour the low-sodium beef broth around it.

4. Cover the dish with aluminum foil and roast in the oven for 1 hour, or until the internal temperature reaches 145°F for medium-rare.

5. While the beef is roasting, steam the cauliflower until tender, about 10-15 minutes.

6. Drain the cauliflower and transfer to a large bowl. Add the unsalted butter and mash until smooth.

7. Remove the roast beef from the oven and let it rest for 10 minutes before slicing.

8. Serve slices of roast beef with a generous portion of mashed cauliflower. Garnish with fresh parsley.

Nutritional Information:

- Calories: 350 per serving
- Protein: 30g
- Carbohydrates: 10g
- Dietary Fiber: 4g
- Sodium: 180mg
- Potassium: 600mg
- Phosphorus: 220mg

Serving Size: 4 ounces of roast beef with 1 cup of mashed cauliflower

Cooking Time: 1 hour and 25 minutes

Lentil Soup with Spinach and Garlic

Ingredient

1 cup dried lentils, rinsed

6 cups low-sodium vegetable broth

1 tablespoon olive oil

1 medium onion, finely chopped

2 cloves garlic, minced

1 cup fresh spinach, chopped

1 teaspoon ground cumin

1/2 teaspoon ground turmeric

1/2 teaspoon ground black pepper

1/2 teaspoon dried thyme

1 bay leaf

Juice of 1 lemon

Instructions

1. In a large pot, heat olive oil over medium heat. Add the chopped onion and minced garlic, sautéing until the onion is translucent.

2. Add the rinsed lentils, vegetable broth, ground cumin, ground turmeric, ground black pepper, dried thyme, and bay leaf to the pot. Stir to combine.

3. Bring the mixture to a boil, then reduce the heat and let it simmer for about 25-30 minutes, or until the lentils are tender.

4. Stir in the chopped spinach and lemon juice. Cook for an additional 5 minutes until the spinach is wilted and incorporated into the soup.

5. Remove the bay leaf before serving. Adjust seasoning to taste if necessary.

Nutritional Information

Calories: 220 per serving

Protein: 12g

Carbohydrates: 35g

Fiber: 15g

Sodium: 90mg

Potassium: 350mg

Phosphorus: 200mg

Serving Size

Serves 4

Cooking Time

40 minutes

Stuffed Bell Peppers without Tomato Sauce

Ingredient:

- 4 large bell peppers (any color)
- 1 cup cooked white rice
- 1/2 pound lean ground turkey
- 1 small onion, finely chopped
- 1 small zucchini, finely chopped
- 1/2 cup shredded carrots
- 1/4 cup chopped fresh parsley
- 1 teaspoon dried oregano
- 1 teaspoon garlic powder
- 1/2 teaspoon black pepper
- 1/4 cup low-sodium chicken broth
- 1/4 cup shredded low-fat mozzarella cheese

Instructions:

1. Preheat the oven to 375°F (190°C).
2. Cut the tops off the bell peppers and remove the seeds and membranes.
3. In a large skillet, cook the ground turkey over medium heat until browned.
4. Add the onion, zucchini, and shredded carrots to the skillet and cook until the vegetables are tender.

5. Stir in the cooked rice, parsley, oregano, garlic powder, and black pepper.

6. Remove from heat and spoon the mixture into the bell peppers.

7. Place the stuffed peppers in a baking dish and pour the chicken broth around the base of the peppers.

8. Cover the dish with aluminum foil and bake for 25 minutes.

9. Remove the foil, sprinkle the peppers with shredded mozzarella cheese, and bake for an additional 10 minutes until the cheese is melted and the peppers are tender.

10. Let cool slightly before serving.

Nutritional Information (per serving):

- Calories: 200
- Protein: 14g
- Carbohydrates: 18g
- Fat: 8g
- Sodium: 150mg
- Potassium: 400mg
- Phosphorus: 150mg

Serving Size:

- 1 stuffed bell pepper

Cooking Time:

- Total: 45 minutes (Preparation: 15 minutes, Cooking: 30 minutes)

Baked Chicken Breast with Seasonal Veggies

Ingredients:

- 2 boneless, skinless chicken breasts (4 oz each)
- 1 tablespoon olive oil
- 1 teaspoon dried rosemary
- 1 teaspoon dried thyme
- 1/2 teaspoon garlic powder
- 1/4 teaspoon black pepper
- 1 cup sliced zucchini
- 1 cup baby carrots
- 1 cup cauliflower florets
- 1/2 lemon, thinly sliced
- 2 tablespoons low-sodium chicken broth

Instructions:

1. Preheat the oven to 375°F (190°C).
2. Place the chicken breasts on a baking sheet lined with parchment paper.
3. Brush the chicken with olive oil and season with rosemary, thyme, garlic powder, and black pepper.
4. Arrange the zucchini, baby carrots, and cauliflower around the chicken breasts.
5. Top the chicken and veggies with lemon slices and drizzle with low-sodium chicken broth.

6. Cover the baking sheet with aluminum foil and bake for 25 minutes.

7. Remove the foil and bake for an additional 10 minutes or until the chicken is cooked through and the vegetables are tender.

8. Let the chicken rest for a few minutes before serving.

Nutritional Information:

- Calories: 280 per serving
- Protein: 28g
- Carbohydrates: 12g
- Dietary Fiber: 4g
- Sugars: 5g
- Fat: 12g (including 2g saturated fat)
- Sodium: 140mg
- Potassium: 650mg
- Phosphorus: 250mg

Serving Size:

- 1 chicken breast with 1 cup of mixed vegetables

Cooking Time:

- Total: 35 minutes (Prep: 10 minutes, Cook: 25 minutes)

Chapter 4: Snacks and Beverages

Safe Snacking Options

Ingredients:

- 2 plain rice cakes

- 1 small apple, thinly sliced

- 1 teaspoon ground cinnamon

- 1 tablespoon honey (optional)

Instructions:

1. Place the rice cakes on a plate.

2. Arrange the apple slices evenly on top of the rice cakes.

3. Sprinkle ground cinnamon over the apple slices.

4. Drizzle with honey if desired.

Nutritional Information:

- Calories: 120 per serving

- Sodium: 10 mg

- Potassium: 75 mg

- Phosphorus: 15 mg

- Protein: 1 g

Serving Size: 2 rice cakes

Cooking Time: 5 minutes

Cucumber Dill Dip

Ingredients:

- 1 cup Greek yogurt (low-fat, unflavored)
- 1/2 cucumber, finely chopped
- 1 teaspoon dried dill
- 1 clove garlic, minced
- 1 tablespoon lemon juice
- Salt to taste (use a kidney-friendly salt substitute if available)

Instructions:

1. In a bowl, mix Greek yogurt, cucumber, dill, garlic, and lemon juice.
2. Add salt substitute to taste and stir well.
3. Chill in the refrigerator for at least 30 minutes before serving with low-sodium crackers.

Nutritional Information:

- Calories: 50 per serving
- Sodium: 30 mg
- Potassium: 100 mg
- Phosphorus: 80 mg
- Protein: 5 g

Serving Size: 1/4 cup

Cooking Time: 10 minutes (plus chilling time)

Herbal Iced Tea

Ingredients:
- 4 cups water
- 4 herbal tea bags (such as chamomile or mint)
- 1 tablespoon honey (optional)
- Lemon slices for garnish

Instructions:
1. Boil the water and remove from heat.
2. Steep the tea bags in the hot water for 5-7 minutes.
3. Remove the tea bags and let the tea cool to room temperature.
4. Sweeten with honey if desired and chill in the refrigerator.
5. Serve over ice with lemon slices for garnish.

Nutritional Information:
- Calories: 20 per serving
- Sodium: 0 mg
- Potassium: 10 mg
- Phosphorus: 0 mg
- Protein: 0 g

Serving Size: 1 cup

Cooking Time: 15 minutes

Recommended Beverages

Herbal Lemon Iced Tea

-Ingredients:

- 4 cups water
- 2 herbal tea bags (caffeine-free)
- 1 lemon, thinly sliced
- 1 tablespoon honey (optional)

Instructions:

- Boil water and steep the tea bags for 5 minutes.
- Remove the tea bags and let the tea cool.
- Add lemon slices and honey if desired.
- Refrigerate until cold and serve over ice.

Nutritional Information:

- Calories: 10 (without honey), 40 (with honey)
- Sodium: 0 mg
- Potassium: 30 mg
- Phosphorus: 5 mg

- **Serving Size:** 1 cup

- **Cooking Time:** 10 minutes (plus chilling time)

Cucumber Mint Water

Ingredients:

- 4 cups water
- 1 cucumber, thinly sliced
- 10 fresh mint leaves

Instructions:

- Combine water, cucumber slices, and mint leaves in a pitcher.
- Refrigerate for at least 2 hours to infuse flavors.
- Serve chilled.

Nutritional Information:

- Calories: 5
- Sodium: 0 mg
- Potassium: 15 mg
- Phosphorus: 5 mg

Serving Size: 1 cup

Cooking Time: 5 minutes (plus chilling time)

Cinnamon Apple Water

- Ingredients:
  - 4 cups water
  - 1 apple, thinly sliced
  - 1 cinnamon stick

Instructions:

- Combine water, apple slices, and cinnamon stick in a pitcher.
- Refrigerate for at least 2 hours to infuse flavors.
- Serve chilled.

Nutritional Information:

- Calories: 10
- Sodium: 0 mg
- Potassium: 20 mg
- Phosphorus: 5 mg

Serving Size: 1 cup

Cooking Time: 5 minutes (plus chilling time)

Conclusion

The "Stage 3 Kidney Disease Diet Cookbook for Seniors" is a vital resource for those navigating the complexities of kidney disease management. As we have explored, the dietary adjustments necessary for managing Stage 3 kidney disease can be daunting, but this cookbook makes the process more accessible and less intimidating. By providing a wide array of recipes that are both nutritious and tailored to the specific needs of seniors with kidney disease, this cookbook becomes more than just a guide—it becomes a lifeline.

The cookbook's thoughtful design, with easy-to-read print and simple instructions, ensures that seniors can independently or with minimal assistance prepare meals that support their health. This sense of independence is crucial for maintaining dignity and quality of life. Furthermore, the comprehensive approach, which includes meal planning tips and shopping guides, offers a practical and supportive framework for both seniors and their caregivers.

The focus on balancing essential nutrients, such as managing protein intake, reducing sodium, potassium, and phosphorus, and ensuring adequate hydration, is meticulously addressed in the recipes. This careful consideration helps to alleviate the burden on the kidneys and supports overall health. The inclusion of snacks and beverages that adhere to these guidelines provides variety and ensures that seniors can enjoy a diverse and satisfying diet without compromising their health.

This cookbook also serves as an educational tool, helping seniors and their families understand the importance of each dietary choice. By explaining how certain ingredients benefit kidney health and why others should be limited, the cookbook empowers users with knowledge that fosters informed decision-making and promotes long-term health management.

Incorporating this cookbook into daily routines can lead to significant health improvements. Many users, like Grandpa Joe, experience stabilized kidney function, better energy levels, and an improved sense of well-being. These benefits are not just physical; they enhance mental and emotional health by reducing the stress and anxiety associated with dietary restrictions and health management.

Ultimately, the "Stage 3 Kidney Disease Diet Cookbook for Seniors" stands out as an essential resource for anyone dealing with Stage 3 kidney disease. It provides practical, actionable solutions that make a significant difference in managing the condition. The combination of expert nutritional guidance, easy-to-follow recipes, and educational content makes it an invaluable addition to any senior's health regimen.

By integrating this cookbook into their lives, seniors with Stage 3 kidney disease can take proactive steps towards better health, enjoying delicious meals that support their dietary needs while maintaining the pleasure of eating well. It is a testament to the idea that managing kidney disease doesn't have to be a struggle—it can be a journey towards a healthier, more fulfilling life.

www.ingramcontent.com/pod-product-compliance
Lightning Source LLC
Chambersburg PA
CBHW050826250726
48653CB00006B/2445